The Original Mediterranean Diet Cookbook

Delicious and Healthy Recipes for Beginners
incl. 30 Days Weight Loss Challenge

[1st Edition]

Oliver Garfield

As one of the world's most popular diets today, the Mediterranean diet doesn't use a strict meal plan. Instead, it focuses on whole foods and exercise. In this cookbook, we are going to give you a nice introduction and some scrumptious recipes you can use to live the Mediterranean lifestyle.

What is the Mediterranean Diet?

The countries surrounding the Mediterranean Sea have very similar eating patterns, and that is what the Mediterranean diet is based off of. You will not find a set bunch of rules, either (although there are some guidelines). The meals prepared for this diet use whole fruits, vegetables, grains, legumes, and olive oils, as well as other healthy fats. You will find that lean proteins, like chicken and pork, will be used regularly, as will fish. You will also use some red meat, but very little compared to the Western diet. You will be able to drink in moderation.

This diet is designed to help reduce your cholesterol, lower heart disease risks, and help you live an all-around healthier and longer life.

How to Get Started

Getting started with the idea that you should base your diet around the healthy habits of the population that lives around the Mediterranean, there are a few ideas that you may want to consider:

- Always focus on whole foods. Eliminate processed foods as much as possible

- Limit your red meat intake. You don't have to cut red meat out of your diet completely, but limiting yourself to a couple of times a month is a great idea.

- Cook with olive oil whenever you can. Olive oil is the main fat source in the Mediterranean, and it is a healthy fat.

- Reduce your dairy consumption. Limit the amount of cheese and milk-based products. Use yogurt as a substitute whenever you can.

- Get rid of refined grains. Replace your pasta and rice with items like quinoa and bulgur. Whole grains are a big part of the food of the Mediterranean, because they are rich in fiber and vitamin B.

- Nuts are great snacks. They are rich in omega fatty acids, protein and fiber. Snacking on nuts with fruits or vegetables will help you stay full longer.

Now that you are armed with some great tips, it is time to share with you some great recipe options that will help you build a healthier, happier, and longer life.

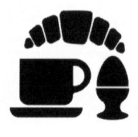

Servings: 2

Nutritional Facts – Calories: 649 | Carbs: 86.4g | Fat: 24.6g | Protein: 23.9g

Ingredients:

- 2 pcs. whole-wheat/multigrain bread
- 8 halved grape tomatoes
- 2 oz. fresh mozzarella balls (approx. 12)
- Basil leaves, freshly torn
- 2 tbsp. balsamic vinegar or glaze
- Salt & pepper

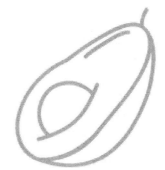

Directions:

1.	Toast the bread to your preferred level of brown. As you are toasting the bread, cut and peel the avocado and put into a small bowl. Then mash until you reach your desired consistency. Add salt and pepper to taste.
2.	Remove the toast from the toaster and spread the avocado on each slice. Once this is done, place the grape tomatoes, mozzarella, and basil over each slice.
3.	Drizzle with balsamic vinegar and serve.

Servings: 4

Nutritional Facts – Calories: 274 | Carbs: 10g | Fat: 18g | Protein: 15g

Ingredients:

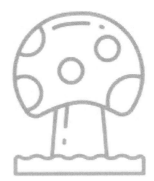

- ◆ 2 eggs
- ◆ 1 tsp. water or milk
- ◆ Kosher salt, 1 pinch
- ◆ Cooking spray (or 1 tbsp. butter)
- ◆ 2 or 3 sliced mushrooms
- ◆ 4-5 trimmed, cut asparagus spears
- ◆ 1 tbsp. green onion, chopped
- ◆ 2 tbsp. goat cheese

Directions:

1.	Set your oven to broil and let it begin the preheating process.
2.	Lightly coat a medium-sized (7 - 8") frying pan with cooking spray. Place on a medium heat and let warm. Once it is heated a little, add mushrooms and sauté until they are slightly soft. Then, add in the asparagus. Cook the asparagus and mushrooms for a few more minutes.
3.	Break the eggs into a small bowl and whisk with the teaspoon of water or milk and a pinch of kosher salt. Continue until the eggs have a nice froth, and the whites and yolk are completely combined.
4.	Pour the egg mixture over the asparagus and mushroom mixture. Top with the goat cheese and green onions. Let cook until the edges begin to brown and pull away from the pan. Lift the eggs gently, tilting the pan to allow for any uncooked egg mixture to begin to cool.
5.	Take a pan and move to the oven. Let the frittata grill for a few minutes. This will finish the cooking process and allow the eggs to puff. When removed from the oven, sprinkle a little more cheese on top. Slice into wedges and serve.

Servings: 4

Nutritional Facts – Calories: 301 | Carbs: 26.5g | Fat: 15.5g | Protein: 15.5g

Ingredients:

- ◆ 3 tbsp. olive oil (divided into individual tbsp.)
- ◆ 15 oz. can of cannellini beans, drained and rinsed
- ◆ 1tsp. kosher salt
- ◆ 2 tsp. za'atar
- ◆ 1 med. bunch, Swiss chard, thinly sliced & stems removed
- ◆ 2 garlic cloves, minced
- ◆ ¼ tsp. crushed red pepper flakes
- ◆ 1 tbsp. lemon juice, freshly squeezed

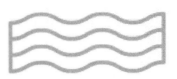

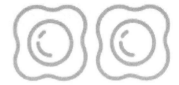

Directions:

1.	Crack each egg into individual cups. Fill the crockpot with water and a teaspoon of vinegar. Let it begin to simmer. Stir the water until there is a whirlpool effect and slowly tip one egg at a time into the center. Cook each egg for 3-4 minutes and then remove gently to a paper towel with a slotted spoon.
2.	Now heat 2 tbsp of oil in the frying pan on medium heat until the oil is hot. Add a can of drained and rinsed cannellini beans. Make sure the beans are spread in an even layer and let cook until the cannellini beans are slightly brown on the bottom.
3.	Add ½ tsp. of salt and 1 tsp. of za'atar and stir. Then spread the beans back out in an even layer and cook until the beans are blistered on the side.
4.	Add the remaining oil to the pan, as well as the chard. Now sprinkle in the remaining salt, the za'atar, garlic, and pepper flakes. Cook until the chard has wilted down. Then remove from the pan and add the lemon juice. Divide the mixture into serving bowls and top with poached egg and, if desired, more crushed pepper flakes.

Servings: 8

Nutritional Facts – Calories: 353 | Carbs: 38.0g | Fat: 20.1g | Protein: 9.3g

Ingredients:

- 1 cup oats, steel-cut
- 1 cup quinoa, dry golden
- ½ cup millet, dry
- 3 tbsp. olive oil
- ¾ tsp. salt
- 1 pc. fresh ginger, peeled and cut into discs
- 2 lrg. Lemons, zest and juice
- ½ cup maple syrup
- 1 cup yogurt, Greek
- ¼ tsp. nutmeg
- 2 cups hazelnuts, toasted and chopped
- 2 cups blueberries, fresh

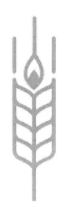

Directions:

1.	Pour and mix the oats, millet, and quinoa into a fine-mesh strainer and wash under cool running water for a minute. Then, set aside to drain.
2.	Over medium-high heat, heat 1 tbsp. of olive oil in a saucepan. Add the rinsed grains and cook for a few minutes, until they begin to smell toasted. Now, add 4 ½ cups of water, along with ¾ tsp. of salt, the ginger, and the zest of 1 lemon.
3.	Bring mixture to a boil, cover with a lid, and turn down heat. Let simmer for 20 minutes. Turn off heat and remove. Leave standing for 5 minutes. Then, remove the lid and use a fork to fluff the mixture. Take out the ginger coins. Now, take the mixture and spread it out over a baking sheet. Leave to cool for about 30 minutes. Once it has cooled, spoon into large bowl and mix in the zest of the lemon.
4.	Combine in medium-sized bowl with 2 tbsp. of olive oil and the juice of two lemons. Whisk until emulsified. Add in maple syrup, yogurt, and nutmeg, and whisk until completely combined. Then, pour over the grain mixture and stir until coated. Add in toasted hazelnuts and blueberries. Taste and add seasonings as desired.
5.	Let sit in the refrigerator overnight and enjoy.

Servings: 8

Nutritional Facts – Calories: 275 | Carbs: 36.4g | Fat: 13.0g | Protein: 8.5g

Ingredients:

- 3 ½ cups oats, rolled
- ½ cup wheat bran
- ½ tsp. salt, kosher
- ½ tsp. cinnamon, ground
- ½ cup almonds, sliced
- ¼ cup pecans, chopped
- ¼ cup pepitas
- ½ cup coconut flakes, unsweetened
- ¼ cup apricots, dried, chopped
- ¼ cup cherries, dried

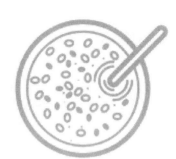

Directions:

1.	Start by toasting the grains, seeds, and nuts. Preheat oven to 350°F and make sure the two racks are evenly distributed. Place the grains on one baking sheet with the salt and cinnamon. Evenly spread nuts and seeds on another baking sheet. Place both baking sheets in the oven and bake until you can smell the nuts. This usually takes 10 – 12 minutes.
2.	Remove baking sheet with the nuts and allow to cool. Pull the grain sheet out and add in the coconut and place back in oven. Bake for further five minutes, or until the coconut is lightly browned. Remove from the oven and allow to cool.
3.	Add both baking sheets to large bowl, then toss in dried fruits and combine.
4.	Place mixture in an airtight container that can be stored at room temperature for up to a month.

Servings: 2

Nutritional Facts – Calories: 261.2 | Carbs: 3.8g | Fat: 15.2g | Protein: 26.1g

Ingredients:

- 2 chicken breasts, boneless, skinless
- ¼ cup olive oil
- ¼ cup balsamic vinegar, golden
- ⅛ cup mustard, whole grain
- 1 ½ tbsp. balsamic vinegar
- 3 garlic cloves, minced
- Lemon juice, ½ of one lemon
- ½ tbsp. rosemary, fresh
- ½ tbsp. thyme, fresh
- ½ tbsp. basil, fresh
- 1 tsp. salt, kosher
- ½ tsp. pepper, freshly ground
- Feta cheese, chunked

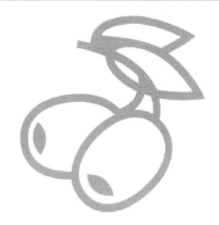

Tapenade

- 3 garlic cloves, minced
- ¼ cup olive oil
- ½ cup sun-dried tomatoes, drained and chopped
- 4 oz. jar green olives, drained and pitted
- 6 oz. jar kalamata olives, drained and pitted
- 1 small jar of capers, drained
- Lemon juice, fresh (whole lemon)
- 2 tsp. balsamic vinegar
- ½ tsp. pepper, freshly ground
- ⅓ cup parsley, fresh, chopped

Directions:

Tapenade Directions

1.	Place the garlic and olive oil into the food processor and run it on high until everything is completely combined. Open the lid and scrape down the sides, then add sun-dried tomatoes and capers. Run through the processor until tomatoes are chopped.
2.	Now, add olives and pulse until olives are coarsely chopped. Add in lemon juice, vinegar, pepper, parsley, and remaining capers. Stir until mixed thoroughly.

Balsamic Chicken Directions

1.	Trim the chicken of any excess fat and place it in a freezer bag.
2.	In a small bowl, combine the olive oil, vinegar, mustard, garlic, lemon juice, herbs, salt, and pepper. Whisk until all Ingredients are mixed well. Reserve half of the mixture and pour the rest into the freezer bag. Leave it to marinate for a minimum of 30 minutes (best if left overnight), turning occasionally.
3.	Heat grill pan and drizzle olive oil into it. Then place the chicken breasts on the grill. Grill for 3 minutes on each side (depending on how thick the breast is, it may need less or more time to cook). This will give the nice grill marks. Then, lower heat and grill for another 5 minutes per side or until you have an internal temp of 165 ☐ F. While cooking the breasts, have a small bowl of the mixture near you so that you can baste the chicken with it.
4.	Remove breasts to a plate and tent with foil for another 5 minutes to allow the juices to redistribute. Then, serve with tapenade and a sprinkle of feta cheese. Finish off with a drizzle of the reserved marinade over the top.

Servings: 4

Nutritional Facts – Calories: 415 | Carbs: 14g | Fat: 24g | Protein: 31g

Ingredients:

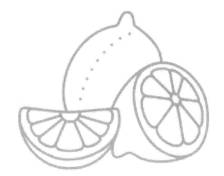

- ◆ 4 pork chops, thin, boneless
- ◆ 8 sage leaves, fresh
- ◆ ¼ cup flour, all-purpose
- ◆ Kosher salt (for taste)
- ◆ Pepper (for taste)
- ◆ 4 tbsp. butter
- ◆ 1 tbsp. vegetable oil
- ◆ ½ cup wine, white
- ◆ ¼ cup capers, drained
- ◆ 1 cup stock, chicken
- ◆ Lemon juice, fresh (2 lemons)
- ◆ 1 lemon, sliced thinly
- ◆ 2 tbsp. parsley, flat-leaf, chopped

Directions:

1.	Pound the pork chops until they are ¼ inch thick. Then, press two sage leaves per chop into the meat.
2.	Combine flour, salt, and pepper in a shallow bowl. Coat the pork chops in the flour, being careful not to dislodge the sage leaves. Carefully remove excess flour.
3.	Heat the skillet over medium heat and melt 1 tbsp. of butter with ½ tbsp. of the oil. Place two of the pork chops into the heated skillet and cook for about 4 minutes per side. Remove and set aside. Add another tbsp. of butter, the remaining oil and repeat the process with the last 2 chops.
4.	Carefully wipe out the skillet to get rid of most of the crispy bits. Then, replace on heat and melt another tablespoon of butter in skillet. Once it is melted, add in the wine and capers. Cook this down until it is reduced by half. Then, add in the stock, lemon juice, and some of the lemon slices. Bring to a boil and then add the rest of the butter into the skillet. Let simmer until the sauce thickens. Then, add chops back into skillet. Let them heat up in the sauce. Serve topped with chopped parsley.

Servings: 4

Nutritional Facts – Calories: 350 | Carbs: 10g | Fat: 7g | Protein: 54g

Ingredients:

- 1 lb. turkey, ground
- ½ cup spinach, fresh, chopped
- ⅓ cup sun-dried tomatoes, chopped
- ¼ cup red onion, minced
- ¼ cup feta, crumbled
- 2 garlic cloves, minced
- 1 egg, whisked
- 1 tbsp. olive oil
- 1 tsp. oregano, dried
- ½ tsp. salt, kosher
- ½ tsp. pepper, freshly ground
- 4 whole-wheat buns
- Lettuce leaves, Bibb
- Red onion, sliced

Tzatziki Ingredients

- ½ cucumber, grated, skin and seeds removed
- ¾ cup Greek yogurt, low-fat
- 2 garlic cloves, minced
- 1 tbsp. red wine vinegar
- 1 tbsp. dill, fresh, minced
- Pinch of kosher salt and pepper

Directions:

1.	Put the ground turkey, spinach, sun-dried tomatoes, red onion and feta in a large bowl. Then, combine garlic, egg, olive oil, oregano, salt, and pepper in small bowl and whisk until thoroughly emulsified. Pour into large bowl with turkey. Mix with your hands and, when completely mixed, divide into four patties. Place on parchment paper that has been laid over a cutting board. Then, refrigerate for at least 30 minutes (overnight is great, as well).
2.	Make the tzatziki sauce. Start by grating the cucumber. Then, place in a paper towel and squeeze to remove the water. Now, you can place it in a small bowl. Add the yogurt, vinegar, dill, garlic, salt, and pepper. Mix until completely combined. Cover the bowl and let stand in refrigerator for at least 30 minutes.
3.	Spray some cooking spray on a grill pan, and heat it over a medium heat
4.	Place turkey burgers on grill pan and cook for about 5 minutes per side. Remove when cooked through and let rest for a minute.
5.	Spread tzatziki on the buns and use the red onion, lettuce, and garnishes for the burger.

Servings: 4

Nutritional Facts – Calories: 322 | Carbs: 28.2g | Fat: 7.2g | Protein: 33.3g

Ingredients:

- ♦ 2 duck breasts
- ♦ Kosher salt and freshly ground black pepper
- ♦ 2 tbsp. pomegranate molasses
- ♦ 2 tbsp. white vermouth
- ♦ 1 lrg. orange, juiced
- ♦ 1 tbsp. honey
- ♦ 1 cinnamon stick
- ♦ 4 cloves, whole
- ♦ ⅛ tsp. cardamom

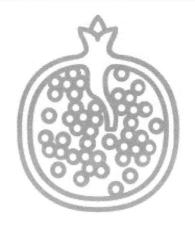

Directions:

1.	Preheat oven to 400°F. Then, on a cutting board, place duck breast fat side up. Use your paring knife to crosshatch the fat. Sprinkle with salt and pepper. Then, place them fat side down into a cold skillet and set the heat to low. Cook them like this for about 12-15 minutes. This renders off the fat.
2.	While the duck is on the stove, combine the molasses, vermouth, orange juice, honey, cinnamon, cloves, and cardamom together in a small saucepan. Bring this up to a simmer and let simmer for about five minutes. Turn off the heat and set to the side.
3.	Once the fat is rendered, drain it from skillet. Save and use later. Now, return duck breasts to pan, fat side up this time. Brush it with the pomegranate syrup you made earlier. Put pan in oven for roughly 5 – 7 minutes.
4.	Once the duck is cooked and the temp reads 160°F, remove it from oven and place on a cutting board. Tent with foil to let rest, but not before you brush it again with the molasses syrup.

Servings: 16

Nutritional Facts – Calories: 70 | Carbs: 4g | Fat: 3g | Protein: 8g

Ingredients:

- ♦ 1 lb. sirloin, boneless, cut 1" thick
- ♦ ½ tsp. garlic powder
- ♦ ½ tsp. black pepper, freshly ground
- ♦ ¼ tsp paprika, smoked

Garlic White Bean Dip

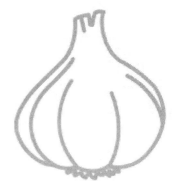

- ♦ 1 can cannellini beans, drained and rinsed
- ♦ 2 tbsp. water
- ♦ 1 tbsp. balsamic vinegar
- ♦ 3 tbsp. olive oil, extra virgin
- ♦ 1 clove garlic, chopped
- ♦ ½ tsp. salt
- ♦ ½ tsp. paprika, smoked

Directions:

1.	Start by making the dip. Place the beans, water, vinegar, 1 tbsp. of olive oil, garlic, and salt into the food processor. Process until smooth. Remove ½ of the dip, sprinkle with paprika, and drizzle 1 tsp. olive oil over the top. Then, place the rest of the dip on top of that and repeat the garnish process. Cover and set aside.
2.	Soak bamboo skewers in water for approximately 10 minutes. While this is soaking, cut the beef into ¼□ thick slices. Then, thread the beef onto the skewers.
3.	Now, combine the garlic, pepper, and paprika into a small bowl and mix until combined. Sprinkle this mixture evenly over the skewers.
4.	Place skewers onto a baking sheet and set oven to broil. Broil the skewers until they are done. Then, serve with dip.

Servings: 6

Nutritional Facts – Calories: 276 | Carbs: 8g | Fat: 6.1g | Protein: 45g

Ingredients:

- 1 lb. chicken breast, boneless, skinless
- ⅓ cup plain yogurt, Greek
- ¼ cup olive oil
- 4 lemons, juiced (1 zested)
- 5 garlic cloves, minced
- 2 tbsp. oregano, dried
- 1 tsp. kosher salt
- ½ tsp pepper, freshly ground
- 1 red onion, quartered 1" pcs.
- 1 zucchini, sliced ¼" pcs.
- 1 red bell pepper, cut into 1" pcs.

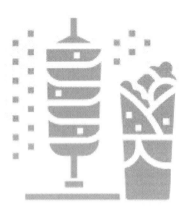

Directions:

1.	Cut chicken breasts into 1" pieces and place it in a freezer bag. Set aside.
2.	Now, combine the Greek yogurt and olive oil into a medium bowl. Then, zest one whole lemon into the bowl and add the juice of lemon, as well. Now, add in the garlic, oregano, salt, pepper, and then mix well. Place half of the marinade into the freezer bag with the chicken. Cover and refrigerate the other half for use when cooking the chicken kebabs. Let chicken and marinade stand for at least 30 minutes.
3.	Oil the grill pan (or grill). Soak your wooden skewers if using wood. Then, cut up the peppers, zucchini, and onion.
4.	Now, it is time to assemble. Alternate vegetables and chicken until your skewer is full. Repeat the process until all your skewers are full.
5.	Heat the grill pan (or grill) and then grill the skewers, using the remaining marinade to baste as you do so. Cook until the chicken juices run clear.

Servings: 4

Nutritional Facts – Calories: 294 | Carbs: 9g | Fat: 17g | Protein: 25g

Ingredients:

- 2 chicken breasts, boneless, skinless
- ½ tsp. salt
- ½ tsp. pepper, ground
- ¼ cup whole wheat flour, white
- 3 tbsp. olive oil, extra virgin
- ½ cup cherry tomatoes, halved
- 2 tbsp. shallots, sliced
- ¼ cup balsamic vinegar
- 1 cup chicken broth, low sodium
- 1 tbsp. garlic, minced
- 1 tbsp. fennel seeds, toasted and crushed
- 1 tbsp. butter

Directions:

1.	Cut each chicken breast in half horizontally. Then, lay on cutting board and place plastic wrap over the breasts. Pound the chicken breasts with the solid side of a meat tenderizer until ¼" thick. Remove the plastic wrap and sprinkle with 1/4tsp. each of salt and pepper on both sides. Then, place the flour in a shallow bowl. Dredge cutlets in flour, making sure to remove excess flour.
2.	In a large skillet, heat 2 tbsp. of oil over a medium heat. Add two pieces of chicken, turning only once, and cook until evenly browned (about two to three minutes). Remove and repeat this process with the other two slices.
3.	Once the chicken is removed, add the rest of the oil, tomatoes, and shallots to skillet. Cook until soft and then add the vinegar. Bring to a boil and scrape all the browned bits from the bottom of the skillet. Once the vinegar is reduced by half, add in the broth, fennel, and the rest of the salt and pepper. Cook while stirring continuously until the sauce is reduced by half. Then, remove from stove, add butter, and serve the sauce over the chicken.

Servings: 4

Nutritional Facts – Calories: 540 | Carbs: 61g | Fat: 24g | Protein: 36g

Ingredients:

- 2 spaghetti squash
- 1 lb. ground turkey, lean
- 1 onion, diced
- 4 garlic cloves, minced
- 14 oz. canned diced tomatoes, Italian-style
- 2 cups mushrooms, sliced
- 6 oz. spinach
- 1 tsp. thyme
- 1 tsp. rosemary
- 1 tsp. basil, dried
- Salt and pepper
- 1 cup feta cheese

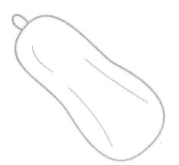

Directions:

1.	Preheat the oven to 400°F. Cut the spaghetti squash lengthwise and scoop out all the seeds. Sprinkle salt and pepper over the meat of the squash. Then, bake for 1 hour with the flesh side down.
2.	Heat a skillet over a medium heat and add the turkey and onion into it. Cook until browned. Then, break the turkey up into little pieces and add garlic. Cook until the garlic is fragrant.
3.	Next, add in the diced tomatoes (juice and all), mushrooms, spinach, thyme, rosemary, and dried basil. Bring this mixture up to a simmer and let it simmer while the spaghetti squash is baking. Taste and add seasonings if needed.
4.	Once spaghetti squash is cooked, scoop out spaghetti squash and add to mixture.
5.	Spray casserole dish and add the mixture into the dish. Top with feta and bake for 10 minutes.

Nutritional Facts – Calories: 230 | Carbs: 9g | Fat: 9g | Protein: 28g

Ingredients:

- 8 pork chops, thin, boneless
- 1 sm. zucchini
- 1 sm. yellow squash
- 1 cup grape tomatoes, halved
- 1 tbsp. olive oil, extra-virgin
- ¼ tsp. kosher salt and pepper
- ¼ tsp. oregano
- 3 garlic cloves, sliced thin
- Cooking spray
- ¼ cup kalamata olives, pitted and sliced
- ¼ cup feta, crumbled
- Lemon juice fresh (half a lemon)
- 1 tsp. lemon rind, zested
- Seasoning Ingredients
- ⅛ tsp. garlic powder
- ⅛ tsp. onion powder
- ⅛ tsp. lemon pepper
- ⅛ tsp. parsley flakes
- ⅛ tsp. coriander, ground
- ⅛ tsp. pepper
- ⅛ tsp. paprika
- ⅛ tsp. turmeric

Directions:

1.	In a small bowl, combine the Ingredients for the seasoning. Mix well. Then, preheat the oven to 450°F. Season the pork chops with the seasoning mixture.
2.	Cut the zucchini and yellow squash into matchsticks (or use your mandolin). Then, in a bowl, toss the grape tomatoes with ½ tbsp. of oil, salt, pepper, and oregano. Spread the tomatoes onto a baking sheet and roast in the oven for 10 minutes, adding the garlic slices about halfway through. Once this is done, return mixture to the bowl and set to the side.
3.	Reduce heat in the oven to 200°F. Then, heat skillet and add ½ tablespoon of oil, zucchini, squash, and salt. Sauté until tender and then add to tomatoes and place in oven to keep warm.
4.	Cook the pork chops in batches over a medium heat for about 2 minutes per side. Then, remove vegetables from oven and add the lemon juice, lemon rind, and kalamata olives. Serve over the pork chops with feta cheese crumbled on top.

Servings: 4

Nutritional Facts – Calories: 280 | Carbs: 11g | Fat: 13g | Protein: 28g

Ingredients:

- 2 steaks, strip
- 4 ½ tsp. garlic, minced
- 1 cup red onion, thinly sliced
- 10 ½ oz. grape tomatoes, halved
- 10 oz. baby spinach, fresh

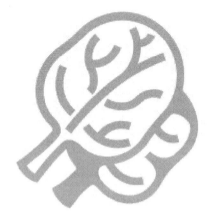

Directions:

1.	Take 2 ½ tsp. of minced garlic and press it evenly into the steaks. Cover them and let them stand in the refrigerator for 30 minutes.
2.	Next, remove and place on a heated grill pan. Grill the steaks until the desired doneness, only turning occasionally.
3.	Now, heat a large skillet and add onion and 2 tsp. of minced garlic. Cook until soft and garlic fragrant. Then, add tomatoes and kalamata olives. Cook these until soft, as well. Then, stir the spinach and take off the heat. The carryover heat will wilt the spinach down.
4.	Once the steak has rested a few minutes, thinly slice it. Serve over the top of the spinach mixture.

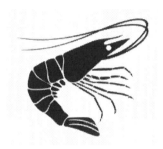

Servings: 4

Nutritional Facts – Calories: 280 | Carbs: 13g | Fat: 15g | Protein: 24g

Ingredients:

- 2 tbsp. olive oil, extra virgin
- 2 garlic cloves, minced
- 1 lb. raw shrimp, peeled and de-veined
- 1 cup chicken broth, low sodium
- 1 tbsp. cornstarch
- ⅓ cup white wine
- ¼ cup lemon juice, fresh
- 3 tbsp. capers, drained and rinsed
- 2 tbsp. parsley, fresh, chopped

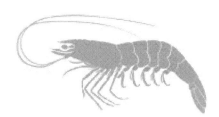

Directions:

1.	Cut the zucchini lengthwise and use your spiralizer or peeler to cut into noodles. Stop when you get to the seeds. Put noodles in colander and toss with salt. Let drain for 15 - 30 minutes. Then, squeeze out excess water.
2.	Heat butter and 1 tbsp. oil in a skillet over medium heat. Add in the garlic and cook until fragrant. Then, add shrimp and cook, stirring for one minute.
3.	Combine broth and cornstarch in a small bowl and whisk until combined. Add shrimp and then add the wine, lemon juice, and capers. Simmer, stirring occasionally until the shrimp is cooked all the way. Then, remove from heat.
4.	Heat 1 tbsp. of the oil in a skillet over medium heat and add in the zucchini noodles. Toss until hot. Then, serve with shrimp and sauce over the noodles sprinkled with a little parsley.

Servings: 4

Nutritional Facts – Calories: 222 | Carbs: 4g | Fat: 12g | Protein: 24g

Ingredients:

- ◆ 2 tsp. Dijon mustard
- ◆ 1 garlic clove, minced
- ◆ ¼ tsp. lemon zest
- ◆ 1 tsp. rosemary, fresh, chopped
- ◆ ½ tsp. honey
- ◆ ½ tsp. salt
- ◆ ¼ tsp. red pepper flakes
- ◆ 3 tbsp. breadcrumbs, panko
- ◆ 3 tbsp. walnuts, finely chopped
- ◆ 1 tsp. olive oil, extra-virgin
- ◆ 1lb. salmon fillet, fresh or frozen

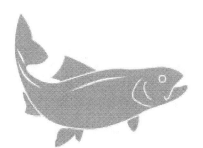

Directions:

1.	Preheat oven to 425°F. Line a baking sheet with parchment paper.
2.	In a small bowl, combine the mustard, zest, juice, rosemary, honey, salt, and red pepper flakes. In another small bowl, combine panko, walnuts, and oil.
3.	Set salmon onto the baking sheet and spread some of the mustard mixture on each piece. Once it's done, you can then top each fillet with the breadcrumb mix. Make sure to press it down gently until it sticks to the fish.
4.	Bake until salmon is flaky (about 8 – 12 minutes).
5.	Sprinkle with parsley and add a lemon wedge when you serve.

Servings: 4

Nutritional Facts – Calories: 241 | Carbs: 7.2g | Fat: 7.8g | Protein: 34.8g

Ingredients:

- 1 lb. large shrimp, peeled and de-veined
- ½ tsp. red pepper flakes
- ¼ tsp. kosher salt
- 3 tbsp. olive oil
- 1 med. onion, chopped
- 3 garlic cloves, minced
- 15 oz. canned crushed tomatoes
- ½ tsp. allspice, ground
- ½ tsp. cinnamon, ground
- ½ cup feta cheese, crumbled
- 2 tbsp. dill, fresh, chopped

Directions:

1.	Preheat oven to 375 ☐ F. Then, rinse and dry the shrimp. Place the shrimp in a bowl and season with salt, pepper, and pepper flakes.
2.	Heat a heavy skillet with olive oil over medium heat. Then, add in garlic and onion and sauté until soft. Stir in the spice and cook until you smell the spices. Add in the tomatoes and let simmer for 20 minutes.
3.	Take the skillet off the heat and place shrimp into the sauce. Crumble feta over the top. Then, bake for 15 - 18 minutes or until shrimp is fully cooked.
4.	When done, sprinkle with dill. Serve with crusty bread.

Servings: 4

Nutritional Facts – Calories: 577 | Carbs: 38g | Fat: 24g | Protein: 38g

Ingredients:

- 4 bass fillets
- Sea salt
- Herbs de Provence
- 1 tbsp. Dijon mustard
- 3 med. tomatoes, diced
- ⅓ cup olives, mixed, pitted, and chopped
- 1 tbsp. capers
- 1 garlic clove, minced
- 2 tbsp. olive oil
- 1 tbsp. white wine vinegar
- Parsley, chopped - garnish

Directions:

1.	Preheat the broiler.
2.	Rinse fish and pat dry. Place the fish on the baking sheet. Season with salt and herbs de Provence. Spread a generous amount of Dijon mustard on top of each fillet.
3.	Mix together the tomatoes, capers, garlic, olive oil, vinegar and ½ tsp. of salt in a medium bowl. Spoon the mixture over the fish.
4.	Bake fish in the broiler for 10 minutes or until fish is cooked through. Rotate the pan or skillet halfway through.
5.	Garnish with parsley.

Servings: 4

Nutritional Facts – Calories: 226 | Carbs: 44g | Fat: 1g | Protein: 8g

Ingredients:

- 1 cup chicken broth
- 1 ¼ cups couscous
- ¾ tsp. kosher salt
- 2 - 5 oz. cans oil-packed tuna
- 1-pint cherry tomatoes, halved
- ½ cup sliced pepperoncini
- ⅓ cup parsley, fresh, chopped
- ¼ cup capers
- Extra-virgin olive oil, for serving
- Kosher salt and pepper
- 1 lemon, quartered

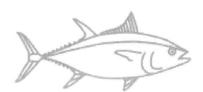

Directions:

1.	Bring the broth to a boil in a small pot. Remove the pot from the heat, add in the couscous, and cover. Leave to stand for 10 minutes.
2.	Combine the tuna, tomatoes, pepperoncini, parsley, and capers together in a medium bowl.
3.	Uncover couscous and fluff it with a fork. Season with salt and pepper and drizzle with olive oil. Top the couscous with the tuna mixture and serve with lemon wedges.

Servings: 4

Nutritional Facts – Calories: 230 | Carbs: 4.6g | Fat: 11.2g | Protein: 27.9g

Ingredients:

- ◆ 4 tilapia fillets
- ◆ ¼ cup basil pesto
- ◆ ½ cup parmesan cheese, freshly grated
- ◆ 1 cuptomatoes, chopped
- ◆ Salt, pepper, lemon juice, melted butter

Directions:

1.	Preheat the broiler. Pat the tilapia dry with a paper towel. Then, place each fillet onto a foil-lined baking sheet. Coat the fillet with oil before doing this to keep the fish from sticking.
2.	Sprinkle each fillet with 2 tbsp. of parmesan cheese. Broil for 10-11 minutes or until the fish is cooked through.
3.	Top each fillet with fresh tomatoes and pesto. You can also top with salt, pepper, lemon juice, and melted butter.

Servings: 5

Nutritional Facts – Calories: 523 | Carbs: 23g | Fat: 31g | Protein: 41g

Ingredients:

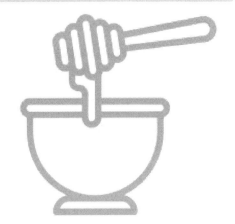

- 1 tbsp. raw honey
- 1 tbsp. coarse-grained mustard
- ½ tsp. white wine vinegar
- Sea salt and black pepper
- 1 - 2lb. salmon fillet
- 2 ½ cups butternut squash, peeled, seeded, and cubed
- 12 oz. Brussel sprouts, trimmed and halved
- 2 cups cherry tomatoes
- 2 tbsp. avocado oil
- ½ tsp. lemon juice, fresh
- ¼ tsp. garlic powder
- ¼ tsp. onion powder
- ¾ tsp. oregano, dried
- ⅛ tsp. turmeric, ground
- 1 lemon, thinly sliced

Directions:

1.	Combine in a small bowl the honey, mustard, vinegar, ½ tsp. of oregano, ½ tsp. salt, and ¼ tsp. pepper and whisk until it is thoroughly mixed. Place the fillets in a baking dish and pour the marinade over the fish. Marinate for 15 minutes.
2.	Preheat oven to 400°F. Then, in a large bowl combine squash, Brussel sprouts, tomatoes, oil, lemon juice, garlic powder, onion powder, the rest of the oregano, turmeric, salt, and pepper. Toss the vegetables until fully coated and then spread out on a baking sheet.
3.	Remove the fish from the marinade and place it in the center of baking sheet. Keep excess marinade to baste while cooking. Roast the fish until it is flaky and the veggies are crispy, yet tender.

Servings: 4

Nutritional Facts – Calories: 186 | Carbs: 6g | Fat: 16g | Protein: 6g

Ingredients:

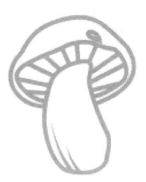

- ◆ 1 garlic clove, minced
- ◆ ½ tsp. salt
- ◆ ½ tsp. pepper
- ◆ 4 portobello mushrooms, stems and gills removed
- ◆ 1 cup cherry tomatoes, halved
- ◆ ½ cup mozzarella pearls
- ◆ ½ cup basil, fresh, sliced
- ◆ 2 tsp. balsamic vinegar

Directions:

1.	Preheat the oven to 400°F. Then, combine 2 tbsp. of oil with garlic, ¼ tsp. salt, and ¼ tsp. pepper in a small bowl. Use a brush to coat the mushrooms. Next, place on a baking sheet and bake until soft.
2.	In a medium bowl, combine the tomatoes, mozzarella, basil, salt, pepper, and oil. Fill the mushrooms with the mixture and bake for a further 12 minutes. Drizzle each mushroom with vinegar and serve.

Servings: 6

Nutritional Facts – Calories: 324 | Carbs: 19g | Fat: 21g | Protein: 17g

Ingredients:

- ¼ tsp. salt
- 2 cups crushed tomatoes
- 1 tsp. Italian seasoning
- 4 tsp. garlic, minced
- ¼ tsp. crushed red pepper flakes
- 2 ½ cups ricotta cheese, part-skim
- ¼ cup parmesan cheese, grated
- ½ tsp. pepper
- ¼ cup almonds, chopped

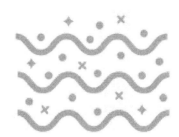

Directions:

1.	Preheat oven to 425°F. Spray two baking sheets with cooking spray.
2.	Slice each zucchini lengthwise into 1/8" thick strips. Brush the strips with oil and sprinkle with salt. Place on one of the baking sheets and roast until soft. Then, reduce heat to 350 ☐F.
3.	Mix tomatoes, Italian seasoning, 2 tsp. garlic and crushed red peppers in a large bowl. Then, spread that mix into a baking dish.
4.	Next, add the ricotta, parmesan, pepper, and garlic in another bowl. Once the zucchini is cool, spoon the ricotta into each slice and roll up and place seam down in the baking dish. Bake for 25-30 minutes.
5.	While this is in the oven, put the almonds and the rest of the garlic, as well as some salt, into a food processor. Process until coarsely ground. Heat a bit of oil in a skillet and add the almond mix into it. Cook until it is fragrant and slightly browned. Serve as a topping.

Servings: 4

Nutritional Facts – Calories: 427 | Carbs: 60.9g | Fat: 16.5g | Protein: 13.2g

Ingredients:

- 4 lrg. sweet potatoes, washed and dried
- 2 tbsp. olive oil
- 1 sm. yellow onion, finely chopped
- ½ tsp kosher salt
- 15 oz. can black beans, drained and rinsed
- ¼ cup water
- 1 can chipotle in adobo chili, finely chopped
- 3 tsp. adobo sauce
- 1 med. lime, halved
- ½ cup Greek yogurt, whole-milk, plain

Directions:

1.	Line a baking sheet with aluminum foil. Stab the sweet potatoes with a fork in multiple spots. Spread on the baking sheet and bake until tender (about 1 hr.). Now, you can make the chipotle black beans.
2.	Heat the oil in a skillet over medium heat. Then add in the onion and cook until soft and translucent. Sprinkle in salt.
3.	Add the beans, water chipotle chile, and 1 tbsp. adobo sauce. Cover and let simmer for several minutes. Do this until the water has evaporated from the mixture. Remove from heat and take half a lime and squeeze into the mixture.
4.	Now, mix yogurt with the remaining adobo sauce in a small bowl.
5.	Once the potatoes are cooked, cut down the center and fill with black beans. Top with avocado, yogurt, and cilantro. Squeeze some lime juice over the top and serve.

Servings: 4

Nutritional Facts – Calories: 324 | Carbs: 27g | Fat: 21g | Protein: 9g

Ingredients:

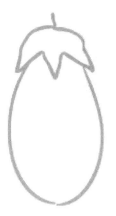

- ♦ 2 sm. eggplants
- ♦ 2 tbsp. olive oil, extra-virgin
- ♦ 2 garlic cloves, chopped
- ♦ ¼ tsp. salt
- ♦ ½ tsp. ground pepper
- ♦ ½ cup parmesan cheese, finely grated
- ♦ 1 ¼ cup breadcrumbs
- ♦ 1 large egg, lightly beaten
- ♦ ⅓ cup parsley, fresh chopped
- ♦ 1 tsp. capers, rinsed
- ♦ 1 ¼ cups tomato sauce
- ♦ 4 lrg. basil leaves

Directions:

1.	Preheat the oven to 375°F. Then, halve the eggplant lengthwise. Trim off a bit of underside to allow them to lay flat. Cut around the inside edge with a paring knife and separate the flesh from the skin. Scoop out the flesh and roughly chop. Set the shells aside.
2.	In a medium saucepan over medium heat, warm 2 tbsp. of oil. Then, add in the meat of the eggplant and cook until soft. Add in the garlic and cook until fragrant. Move this to a bowl and season with salt and pepper. Let cool.
3.	Heat ¼ cup of oil in the skillet. Season shells with salt, pepper, and 2 tbsp. of parmesan. Then, cook the shells until golden brown and soft. Drain on paper towels.
4.	Dunk breadcrumbs in water and then squeeze them out. Place them in the bowl with the eggplant filling. Then add ¼ cup parmesan, egg, parsley, and capers. Mix well. Fill the eggplant shells with the stuffing.
5.	Spread the tomato sauce on the bottom of a baking dish and then place the stuffed shells in the dish, as well. Spoon some of the sauce over the shells and top with a basil leaf. Sprinkle some parmesan on top. Bake until it is hot, about 25 minutes.

Servings: 6 - 8

Nutritional Facts – Calories: 292 | Carbs: 47.5g | Fat: 6.8g | Protein: 12.8g

Ingredients:

- 4 med. carrots, peeled and sliced
- 2 celery stalks, sliced
- 1 lrg. onion, chopped
- ½ sm. head savoy cabbage, chopped
- 3 garlic cloves, minced
- 2- 15 oz. cans cannellini beans, drained, rinsed
- 14.5 oz. can dice tomatoes
- 6 cups water
- 1 pc. parmesan cheese rind (optional)
- 1 tbsp. kosher salt
- ½ tsp. pepper
- 1 sprig of rosemary, fresh
- 1 lrg. sprig of thyme, fresh
- 1 sprig of oregano, fresh
- 1 med. zucchini, chopped

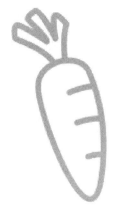

Crouton Ingredients

- 8 oz. country bread, 1" cubes
- 3 tbsp. olive oil
- ½ tsp. kosher salt
- ½ tsp. black pepper
- 1 sprig of rosemary, fresh
- Parsley leaves, fresh chopped
- Red pepper flakes

Directions:

1.	Place all Ingredients except the zucchini in a large crockpot. Cover and cook on low for 6– 8 hours.
2.	Remove the fresh herbs and the parmesan rind. Take 2 cups of soup out and place in blender. Puree herbs and rind and then return it to the soup and mix well. Add the zucchini and cook for a further 30 minutes.
3.	Preheat oven to 400°F. Toss cubed bread in the olive oil, salt, and pepper in a large bowl. Spread out onto a baking sheet in a single layer. Scatter fresh herbs over the bread. Bake until the croutons are golden brown.
4.	When the soup is done, use it to garnish as you serve.

WESTERN-STYLE BREAKFAST BURRITOS

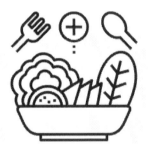

Servings: 4

Nutritional Facts – Calories: 164 | Carbs: 11.6g | Fat: 11.8g | Protein: 5.4g

Ingredients:

- 2 cups arugula, fresh
- 2-3 tomatoes, sliced
- ½ avocado, pitted and sliced
- 3 slices mozzarella cheese, fresh
- Basil leaves, fresh
- 1 tbsp. olive oil, extra-virgin
- 1 ½ tsp. balsamic vinegar
- Pinch of salt
- Dollop of honey
- Salt and pepper to taste

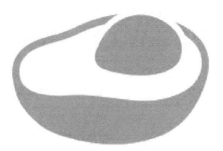

Directions:

1.	Combine together the arugula, tomato, avocado slices, and mozzarella in a serving bowl. Tear basil leaves and top the salad.
2.	In a separate bowl, add in the olive oil, balsamic vinegar, sugar, honey, salt, pepper and whisk until emulsified. Coat salad to your taste and serve.

Servings: 4

Nutritional Facts – Calories: 340 | Carbs: 44.4g | Fat: 13.7g | Protein: 12.1g

Ingredients:

- 2 - 15 oz. cans chickpeas, rinsed, drained
- 1 med. red bell pepper, chopped
- 1 ½ cupsparsley, fresh, chopped
- ½ cup celery plus leaves, chopped
- ½ cup red onion, chopped
- 3 tbsp. olive oil, extra-virgin
- 3 tbsp. fresh lemon juice
- 2 garlic cloves, minced
- ½ tsp. kosher salt and black pepper

Directions:

1.	In the serving bowl, add chickpeas, bell pepper, parsley, red onion, and celery.
2.	Then, in a separate bowl, add olive oil, lemon juice, garlic, salt, pepper and whisk until emulsified. Dress salad and serve.

Servings: 4

Nutritional Facts – Calories: 327 | Carbs: 40g | Fat: 12g | Protein: 10g

Ingredients:

- ⅓ cup pine nuts, shelled
- 1 tbsp. olive oil
- ½ tsp. kosher salt
- 1 ½ cup couscous
- ⅓ cup sun-dried tomatoes in oil, drained and diced
- ⅓ cup feta cheese, crumbled
- ¼ cup green onion, chopped

Directions:

1.	Heat the skillet over medium-high heat and toss in the pine nuts. Toast tossing frequently until golden brown.
2.	In a medium saucepan, boil 1¼ cup water. Stir in couscous, olive oil, and salt. Remove from heat. Cover and let stand.
3.	Using a fork, fluff the couscous and stir in the remaining Ingredients. Serve at room temperature.

Servings: 8

Nutritional Facts – Calories: 440 | Carbs: 16g | Fat: 40g | Protein: 9g

Ingredients:

- 2 cucumbers, peeled and cut ½" slices
- 1 ½ lbs. med. tomatoes, quartered
- ¼ sm. red onion, thinly sliced
- 1 ½ cups kalamata olives, pitted, halved
- ¼ cup parsley. Italian flat-leaf, chopped
- 2 avocados, pitted and cut into chunks
- 1 cup feta cheese, crumbled
- ½ cup olive oil, extra-virgin
- ½ cup red wine vinegar
- 2 garlic cloves, minced
- 1 tbsp. oregano
- 2 tsp. sugar
- 1 tsp. kosher salt
- 1 tsp. pepper

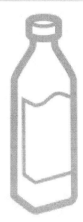

Directions:

1.	In a serving bowl, combine cucumbers, tomatoes, red onion, kalamata olives, and parsley. Place the avocados in a small bowl separate from the rest.
2.	In a small bowl, combine the olive oil, red wine vinegar, garlic, oregano, sugar, salt, and pepper. Whisk until emulsified.
3.	Take 1 tbsp. of dressing and coat the avocados. Pour the rest over the cucumber mixture and coat well. Add the avocado over the salad with feta cheese and serve.

Servings: 2

Nutritional Facts – Calories: 164 | Carbs: 5.7g | Fat: 15.6g | Protein: 3.5g

Ingredients:

- ♦ 2 tbsp. olive oil
- ♦ 2 tbsp. fresh lemon juice
- ♦ 1 tsp. honey
- ♦ ½ tsp. kosher salt
- ♦ ½ tsp. pepper
- ♦ 4 cups arugula
- ♦ ¼ cup parmesan cheese, shaved

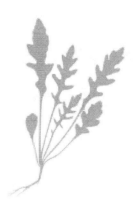

Directions:

| **1.** | In a serving bowl, combine the olive oil, lemon juice, honey, salt, and pepper. Whisk until emulsified. Add the arugula to the bowl and toss. Top with shaved parmesan and add pepper for taste. |

Servings: 12

Nutritional Facts – Calories: 209 | Carbs: 17g | Fat: 18g | Protein: 2g

Ingredients:

- 2 cups coconut, shredded, unsweetened
- ½ cup coconut cream
- 2 tbsp. maple syrup
- 1 tsp. mint extract
- ½ tsp. spirulina
- ¼ cup cocoa nibs
- 1 cup chocolate chips

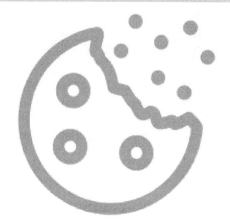

Directions:

1.	In the food processor, add in coconut and process until finely ground. Then, add in the coconut cream, sweetener, mint extract, and spirulina. Process until it all comes together in a sticky dough.
2.	Add the cocoa nibs and blend briefly to mix them.
3.	Scoop with ice cream scoop and shape into cookies. Place in the freezer for 15 minutes until hard. Melt chocolate chips in glass mixing bowl over simmering water. Then, dip frozen cookie in the chocolate. Sprinkle with more cocoa nibs and freeze again until firm.

Servings: 16

Nutritional Facts – Calories: 347 | Carbs: 32g | Fat: 23g | Protein: 7g

Ingredients:

- 2 med. bananas, overripe and smashed
- ¼ cup avocado oil
- ½ cup honey
- 4 eggs
- ¾ cup crushed pineapple
- 2 tsp. vanilla extract
- 3 cups almond flour
- ½ tsp. salt
- 2 tsp. baking soda
- 4 cups coconut whipped cream

Directions:

1.	Preheat oven to 350°F. Grease two 8" cake pans and set to the side.
2.	Combine all Ingredients into a large bowl and mix until thoroughly combined.
3.	Divide batter into each cake pan and smooth the top of the batter.
4.	Bake for 30 – 35 minutes until the top starts to darken and the center is set.
5.	Remove from the oven and let cool. Then, frost with your favorite frosting. Store in refrigerator.

Servings: 4

Nutritional Facts – Calories: 189 | Carbs: 27g | Fat: 7.6g | Protein: 5.9g

Ingredients:

- 1 ¼ cup milk
- 1 cup pumpkin puree
- ½ cup chia seeds
- ¼ cup maple syrup
- 2 tsp. pumpkin spice
- ¼ cup sunflower seeds
- ¼ cup almonds, sliced
- ¼ cup blueberries, fresh

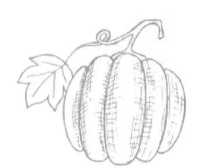

Directions:

| 1. | Add all the Ingredients in a bowl and thoroughly mix. Spoon into canning jars and refrigerate overnight. |
| 2. | Then, serve with either almonds, sunflower seeds, or blueberries. |

Servings: 8

Nutritional Facts – Calories: 26 | Carbs: 1.9g | Fat: 1.9g | Protein: .8g

Ingredients:

♦ 4 zucchini squash, sliced 1/8" rounds

♦ Kosher salt

♦ Olive oil, extra-virgin

♦ Harissa spices

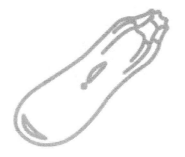

Directions:

1.	Thinly slice the zucchini with a mandolin. Lay out on some paper towels and sprinkle with salt. Then, cover with more paper towels and place a cutting board on top. Let stand for 15 – 20 minutes.
2.	Preheat oven to 245°F. Line the sheet pan with parchment paper and lightly oil with olive oil. Then, lay the zucchini chips out onto the parchment paper in a single layer.
3.	Brush each chip with olive oil and sprinkle with harissa. Bake in the oven for about 2 hours until crisp and golden. Serve with tzatziki at room temperature.

Servings: 1 cup

Nutritional Facts – Calories: 55 | Carbs: 2g | Fat: 4g | Protein: 3g

Ingredients:

- ⅓ cup sun-dried tomatoes, oil-packed
- 2 garlic cloves, halved
- 1 tbsp. basil, fresh, minced
- 1 tbsp. parsley, fresh, minced
- 8 oz. goat cheese, cubed

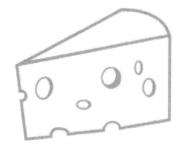

Directions:

| 1. | Drain the sun-dried tomatoes, reserving 2 tsp. of the oil. Combine the garlic, basil, and parsley. Process until combined. |
| 2. | Then, add goat cheese, the sun-dried tomatoes, and oil. Cover and run through process until smooth. Chill until ready to serve. Serve with pita chips or fresh vegetables. |

Breakfast - **Eggs w/ Ratatouille**

Servings: 2

Nutritional Facts – Calories: 226 | Carbs: 20.6g | Fat: 12.5g | Protein: 11.1g

Ingredients:

- 1 tbsp. olive oil
- 1 sm. onion, thinly slice and halved
- 1 garlic clove, minced
- 2 med. zucchini
- 2 med. tomatoes, chopped
- ½ tsp. thyme, fresh
- 1 tsp. paprika
- 1 med. red bell pepper
- Salt and pepper
- 2 lrg. eggs

Directions:

1.	In a large skillet, heat oil on medium heat. Then, add the onion and cook until softened. Add the garlic and cook until fragrant. Once that is done, add the squash and cook until soft and brown. Next, you will add the tomatoes, thyme, and paprika. Then, let simmer until it thickens, about 20 minutes.
2.	While you are doing this, roast the red pepper on the stovetop. Once you have done that, let it cool and remove the core and seeds. Remove skillet from heat and add pepper. Then, salt and pepper to taste. Let the dish cool while frying the eggs. Serve with the egg on top.

Lunch - **Greek Turkey Burger pg.18**

Dinner - **Grilled Balsamic Chicken w/ Olive Tapenade pg.14**

Breakfast - **Avocado Toast Caprese Style pg.5**

Lunch - **Cauliflower Salad w/ Dressing**

Servings: 4

Nutritional Facts – Calories: 165 | Carbs: 20g | Fat: 8g | Protein: 6g

Ingredients:

- 1 med. head cauliflower
- 1 tsp. olive oil
- ½ tsp. kosher salt
- ¼ cup shallot, chopped fine
- 3 tbsp. fresh lemon juice
- 2 tbsp. tahini
- ½ cup parsley, flat-leaf, chopped
- ¼ cup dried cherries, chopped
- 1 tbsp. Mint, fresh, chopped
- 3 tbsp. pistachios, roasted, salted, chopped

Directions:

1.	Grate cauliflower into a large microwaveable bowl. Add in olive oil and ¼ tsp. of salt. Cover with plastic wrap and microwave for 3 minutes. Spread cauliflower over a baking sheet and leave to cool.
2.	In a large mixing bowl, add the chopped shallot and lemon juice. Let sit for several minutes. Then, stir in the tahini. Pour cauliflower into the mixture and toss. Add in parsley, mint, cherries, and ¼ tsp. of salt and combine.
3.	Serve sprinkled with chopped pistachios.

Dinner - **Pork Scaloppini w/ Lemon and Capers pg.16**

Breakfast - **Frittata w/ Asparagus, Mushroom, & Goat Cheese pg.6**
Lunch - **Skewered Beef w/ Garlicky White Bean Sauce pg.22**
Dinner - **Chicken Skillet w/ Bulgur**

Servings: 2

Nutritional Facts – Calories: 369 | Carbs: 21g | Fat: 11.3g | Protein: 45g

Ingredients:

- 4 chicken breasts, boneless, skinless
- ¾ tsp. kosher salt
- ½ tsp. pepper
- 1 tbsp. olive oil
- 1 cup red onion, thinly sliced
- 1 tbsp. garlic, sliced thin
- ½ cup uncooked bulgur

- 2 tsp. oregano, dried, chopped
- 4 cups kale, fresh, chopped
- ½ cup roasted red peppers, jarred, sliced
- 1 cup chicken stock, unsalted
- 2 oz. feta, crumbled
- 1 tbsp. dill fresh, chopped

Directions:

1.	Preheat oven to 400°F. Season chicken breasts with salt and pepper. Heat 1 ½ tsp. of oil in a skillet over medium-high heat. Add chicken to the heated pan and cook until browned on both sides. Remove chicken.
2.	Add leftover oil, onion, and garlic to skillet. Cook until soft and garlic is fragrant. Add bulgur and oregano. Cook until the bulgur is toasted. Add in kale and pepper and cook until kale is wilted. Add stock and ¼ tsp. of both salt and pepper. Bring to a boil and remove from heat.
3.	Place chicken back in skillet, put in the oven and bake until the chicken juices run clear. Remove from oven, sprinkle feta and dill over the top, then serve.

Breakfast - **Spinach Feta Breakfast wrap**

Servings: 4

Nutritional Facts – Calories: 543 | Carbs: 46.5g | Fat: 27.0g | Protein: 28.1g

Ingredients:

- 10 lrg. eggs
- ½ lb. baby spinach
- 4 whole-wheat tortillas
- ½ pint grape tomatoes, halved
- 4 oz. feta cheese, crumbled
- Butter or olive oil
- Salt
- Pepper

Directions:

1.	In a large bowl, combine eggs and whisk until fully incorporated. Heat a large skillet over medium-high heat and add in either butter or olive oil to coat the bottom. When it is hot/melted, pour in the eggs and stir periodically until cooked. Add a pinch of salt and a healthy amount of pepper. Then, remove from pan and set aside.
2.	Clean skillet out and then return to medium-high heat, add more oil/ butter. Add in the spinach and cook until wilted down. Remove from skillet and allow to cool.
3.	Place tortilla on cutting board and add about ¼ of the eggs, spinach, tomatoes, and feta in the middle. Wrap the burrito tight and serve. (You can wrap them in aluminum foil and store them in your freezer in freezer bags, as well.)

Lunch - **Couscous w/ Tuna pg.38**

Dinner - **Pomegranate Citrus Glazed Duck Breast pg.20**

Breakfast - **Poached Egg with Greens & White Beans pg.8**

Lunch - **Shrimp Pasta**

Servings: 8

Nutritional Facts – Calories: 322 | Carbs: 28.5g | Fat: 18.5g | Protein: 12.7g

Ingredients:

- 12 oz. pasta, bow tie
- 1 ½ lbs. shrimp, fresh, peeled, deveined
- ¼ cup butter
- 3 garlic cloves, minced
- 12 oz. jar roasted red peppers, drained, chopped
- 1 cup artichoke hearts, quartered
- ½ cup white wine, dry
- 3 tbsp. capers, drained
- ½ cup whipping cream
- 1 tsp. lemon zest
- 2 tbsp. lemon juice
- ¾ cup feta, crumbled
- 2 oz. pine nuts, toasted
- ¼ cup basil, fresh, torn

Directions:

1.	In the Dutch oven, cook pasta according to instructions. Then, drain and return to Dutch oven and cover to keep warm.
2.	Heat butter in a skillet over medium-high heat and then add garlic. Cook until fragrant, then add shrimp. Cook for 2 minutes, then add in red peppers, artichokes, wine, and capers.
3.	Bring this to a boil, then turn down the heat and let simmer uncovered until the shrimp is cooked thoroughly. Stir in cream, lemon zest, and juice. Let return to boil. Reduce heat and let simmer for another minute.
4.	Combine shrimp mixture with pasta and toss gently.
5.	Serve sprinkled with feta, pine nuts, and basil.

Dinner - **Chicken w/ Tomato and Balsamic Sauce pg.26**

Breakfast - **Start Your Morning Right Grain Salad pg.10**
Lunch - **Stuffed Sweet Potatoes pg.46**
Dinner - **Caprese Chicken**

Servings: 2

Nutritional Facts – Calories: 199 | Carbs: 7.3g | Fat: 16.6g | Protein: 6.8g

Ingredients:

- 2 chicken breasts, boneless, skinless
- Kosher salt and pepper for taste
- 1 tbsp. olive oil, extra-virgin
- 1 tbsp. butter

- 1 jar basil pesto of your choice
- 4 oz. mozzarella, grated
- 1 cup grape tomatoes, halved
- ½ cup balsamic glaze
- ⅓ cup basil, fresh, chopped

Directions:

1.	Preheat oven to 400°F. Slice chicken in half lengthwise and season with salt and pepper on both sides of each breast. Heat skillet with oil and butter over medium-high heat. Then, add the chicken breasts and cook on both sides until lightly browned.
2.	Spoon pesto over the top of each chicken breast and top with grated mozzarella, as well as some tomatoes. Place skillet in oven and let bake for 10-12 minutes until chicken is done. Remove and garnish with basil and balsamic glaze.

Breakfast - **Breakfast Pizza**

Servings: 4

Nutritional Facts – Calories: 337 | Carbs: 33.2g | Fat: 17.6g | Protein: 12.3g

Ingredients:

- 1 lrg. avocado
- 1 tbsp. cilantro, fresh, chopped
- 1 ½ tsp. fresh lime juice
- ⅛ tsp. salt

- ½ lb. pizza dough, pre-made
- 4 lrg. eggs
- 1 tbsp. olive oil
- Hot sauce, for serving

Directions:

1.	Cut the avocado and scoop out the flesh into medium bowl. Add in cilantro, lime juice, and salt. Mash until your desired consistency. Taste and add seasonings to your preference.
2.	Split dough into 4 parts. Flour cutting board and roll each piece into about a 6" pie.
3.	Heat a cast-iron skillet over medium-high heat and then place one pizza crust in the skillet. Cook until the dough is browned, and the surface begins to bubble. Flip and repeat on the other side. Use a spatula to press down if it puffs up. Remove and set aside. Repeat with the other pieces of dough.
4.	Spread avocado mixture evenly over pizza dough.
5.	Heat a small frying pan over medium heat. Fry eggs to your preference and then top pizza with them. Serve hot with/without a drizzle of hot sauce.

Lunch - **Chickpea & Herb Salad pg.55**
Dinner - **Mediterranean Spaghetti Squash w/ Turkey pg.28**

Breakfast - **Easy Muesli pg.12**

Lunch - **Falafel and Tomato Salad**

Servings: 4

Nutritional Facts – Calories: 386 | Carbs: 32g | Fat: 25.1g | Protein: 12g

Ingredients:

- ¼ cup olive oil, extra-virgin
- 2 tbsp. red wine vinegar
- ½ tsp. kosher salt
- ½ tsp. pepper
- 2 lbs. tomatoes, sliced ½"
- 4 cups arugula

- 1 cup cucumber, sliced
- ¾ cup red onion, thinly sliced
- ½ cup mint, fresh, torn
- 4 cooked falafel patties
- 2 oz. feta, crumbled
- ¼ cup pine nuts, toasted

Directions:

1.	Combine the oil, vinegar, salt, and pepper in a large bowl. Whisk until emulsified. Add in tomatoes and toss to coat. Let it stand for a few minutes. Place tomatoes on the serving plate. Reserve rest of vinaigrette.
2.	Add arugula, cucumber, onion, mint, and falafel to the vinaigrette in the bowl. Toss gently. Arrange the falafel mixture over the tomatoes. Sprinkle feta and toasted pine nuts. Drizzle any remaining vinaigrette over the top.

Dinner - **Boneless Pork Chops w/ Vegetables pg.30**

Breakfast - **Eggs w/ Ratatouille pg.68**
Lunch - **Arugula Salad w/ Parmesan pg.59**
Dinner - **Grilled Eggplant Skillet**

Servings: 4

Nutritional Facts – Calories: 397 | Carbs: 20g | Fat: 31g | Protein: 14g

Ingredients:

- 7 tbsp. olive oil
- 14 oz. packaged tofu, extra firm, cubed
- 1 lrg. eggplant, sliced ½" thick
- 28 oz. can tomatoes, whole, peeled, drained and chopped
- 2 garlic cloves, grated

- 1 tsp. oregano, fresh, chopped
- ½ tsp. cinnamon, ground
- ½ tsp. cumin, ground
- ¼ tsp. kosher salt
- ¼ tsp. red pepper flakes
- 3 tbsp. feta, crumbled
- ⅓ cup mint, fresh, chopped

Directions:

1.	Preheat broiler.
2.	In a large oven-safe skillet, heat 2 tbsp. of oil over medium-high heat. Add tofu and cook until browned. Remove tofu and add ¼ cup of oil. Lay eggplant slices in the skillet and cook until brown. Flip and repeat the process. Remove skillet from heat.
3.	Combine tomatoes, garlic, seasoning in a medium bowl. Top the eggplant with the tofu and spoon mixture over the top of that. Drizzle top with olive oil and sprinkle feta.
4.	Place skillet in oven and broil for about 4 minutes. Remove garnish with mint and oregano, then serve.

Breakfast - **Frittata w/ Spinach and Artichoke**

Servings: 4 - 6

Nutritional Facts – Calories: 316 | Carbs: 6.4g | Fat: 25.9g | Protein: 17.9g

Ingredients:

- 10 lrg. eggs
- ½ cup sour cream, full fat
- 1 tbsp. Dijon mustard
- 1 tsp. kosher salt
- ¼ tsp. black pepper

- 1 cup parmesan cheese, grated
- 2 tbsp. olive oil
- 14 oz. can artichoke hearts, drained, dried, and quartered
- 5 oz. baby spinach, fresh
- 2 garlic cloves, minced

Directions:

1.	Preheat oven to 400°F. In a large bowl, combine together the eggs, sour cream, mustard, salt, pepper, and ½ cup parmesan cheese. Whisk until combined thoroughly.
2.	Heat the skillet over medium heat with oil until oil is hot. Then, add in the artichokes and cook until lightly browned. Next, add in spinach and garlic. Toss until spinach is wilted and the liquid is gone.
3.	Spread the mix evenly in one layer across the bottom of the skillet and then add the egg mixture. Sprinkle rest of parmesan over the top. Tilt skillet to make sure the mix is evenly distributed over the vegetables. Cook until the edges of the eggs begin to brown and pull from edge of skillet.
4.	Then, remove from stove and put in the oven. Bake for 12 – 15 minutes more until done. Let cool for a few minutes, then slice and serve.

Lunch - **Cauliflower Salad w/ Dressing pg.69**
Dinner - **Walnut Crusted Salmon pg.35**

Breakfast - **Spinach Feta Breakfast Wrap pg.71**

Lunch - **Chicken Quinoa Bowl**

Servings: 2

Nutritional Facts – Calories: 810 | Carbs: 69.4g | Fat: 50g | Protein: 27.2g

Ingredients:

- 1 chicken breast, boneless, skinless, cubed
- ¼ cup olive oil + 2 tbsp.
- 1 lemon, juiced and zested
- 2 garlic cloves, minced
- 2 tsp. oregano, dried

- 1 ½ tsp. kosher salt
- ¼ tsp pepper
- 1 cup broccoli, roasted
- ½ cup tomatoes, roasted
- 1 cup quinoa, dried
- 1 cup feta, crumbled

Directions:

1.	Preheat oven to 400°F. Coat tomatoes and broccoli with oil, salt, and pepper and spread out over baking sheets. Roast until soft and lightly browned. Take out and let cool.
2.	Slice chicken breast into 1" chunks and place in a freezer bag. Combine olive oil, lemon juice and zest, garlic, oregano, salt, pepper and whisk until fully combined. Add to freezer bag and let marinate for at least 30 minutes.
3.	In a skillet, heat 2 tbsp. of oil over medium-high heat. Add the chicken and cook until brown on all sides. Reduce heat and add the broccoli and tomatoes with more olive oil if need be. Warm all the way through.
4.	Rinse your quinoa while bringing a pan of water to a boil. Add in 1 tsp. of salt and the quinoa. Boil until al dente. Then, drain and fluff. Return to pan and let sit for 5-10 minutes.
5.	Assemble bowls and sprinkle with feta, then serve.

Dinner - **Greek Baked Shrimp pg.36**

Breakfast - **Breakfast Pizza pg.74**

Lunch - **Shrimp Pasta pg.72**

Dinner - **Crock Pot Cacciatore**

Servings: 10

Nutritional Facts – Calories: 90 | Carbs: 7g | Fat: 4g | Protein: 7g

Ingredients:

- 10 chicken thighs, skinless, bone-in
- Kosher salt and pepper to taste
- Olive oil, extra virgin
- 5 garlic cloves, chopped fine
- ½ lrg. onion, chopped
- 28 oz. can crushed tomatoes
- ½ med. bell pepper, green, chopped
- ½ med. bell pepper, red, chopped
- 8 oz. mushrooms, sliced
- 2 sprigs of thyme, fresh
- 2 bay leaves
- ⅓ cup parsley, fresh, chopped
- ½ cup parmesan, grated

Directions:

1.	Season the chicken with salt and pepper liberally. Heat the olive oil in a skillet over a medium-high heat. Add in the seasoned chicken and cook until nicely browned on both sides. Add into the crockpot.
2.	Return skillet to heat and add in a little more oil. Then, toss in the garlic and onion and cook until soft. Add this to the crockpot. Do the same for bell peppers and tomatoes.
3.	Cover and cook in crockpot on low for 8 hours. Remove bay leaves and remove the chicken from the sauce. Pull the meat from the bones and put the meat back into the crockpot, stirring it thoroughly. Add in the parsley. Serve over pasta with parmesan sprinkled on top.

Breakfast - **Smoked Salmon & Poached Eggs on Toast**

Servings: 2

Nutritional Facts – Calories: 471 | Carbs: 41.3g | Fat: 22g | Protein: 27.4g

Ingredients:

- 2 slices of multigrain bread
- ½ lrg. avocado
- ¼ tsp. fresh lemon juice
- Pinch of salt and pepper
- 3 ½ oz. salmon, smoked
- 2 eggs
- 2 slices of tomato
- ¼ cup microgreens

Directions:

1.	Poach eggs. Simmer water in a saucepan with a splash of vinegar. Stir it to create a whirlpool and then drop the egg into the water. Cook for 2-3 minutes and then move carefully with ladle to paper towel. Let stand there while you do the rest.
2.	Cut and scoop out the flesh of half of an avocado into a small bowl. Mash with lemon juice, salt, and pepper.
3.	Toast the bread. Then, spread avocado mixture evenly. Add the smoked salmon and poached egg.
4.	Place the tomato and microgreens on the toast and serve.

Lunch - **Falafel & Tomato Salad pg.75**

Dinner - **Stuffed Portobello Mushroom Caprese Style pg.44**

Breakfast - **Avocado Toast Caprese Style pg.5**

Lunch - **Tuna Melt w/ Olive Salsa**

Servings: 4

Nutritional Facts – Calories: 221 | Carbs: 14g | Fat: 11g | Protein: 16g

Ingredients:

- ⅓ cup green olives, pitted
- 1 tbsp. olive oil, extra-virgin
- 2 tsp. lemon zest
- 3 tbsp. fresh lemon juice
- 2 tbsp. parsley, fresh, chopped
- 1 tbsp. sunflower seeds, toasted
- ¼ tsp. kosher salt
- ¼ tsp. pepper

- ¼ tsp. red pepper flakes
- 5 oz. can tuna, in water, drained
- 2 tbsp. dill, fresh, chopped
- 2 tbsp. Greek yogurt, plain, whole milk
- 1 tsp. Dijon mustard
- 1 ½ oz. mozzarella, grated
- 4 slices whole-grain bread

Directions:

1.	Combine olives, 1 tsp. lemon zest, 1 tbsp. lemon juice, parsley sunflower seed, and pepper flakes and stir well.
2.	Mix tuna, dill, mayonnaise, mustard, 1 tsp. zest, 1 tbsp. juice, salt, and pepper until well combined.
3.	Preheat broiler. Lay out bread and top with tuna mixture. Sprinkle on cheese and broil for 2 minutes. Remove top with olive salsa and serve.

Dinner - **Zucchini Lasagna Rolls pg.45**

Breakfast - **Frittata w/ Asparagus, Mushroom & Goat Cheese pg.6**
Lunch - **Chicken Quinoa Bowl pg.78**
Dinner - **Roasted Salmon w/ Vegetables and Citrus**

Servings: 4

Nutritional Facts – Calories: 390 | Carbs: 21g | Fat: 17g | Protein: 38g

Ingredients:

- 1 ½ lb. salmon fillet
- 2 blood oranges, wedged
- 1 navel orange, wedged
- 1 sm. red onion, wedged
- 1 med. golden beet, sliced 1/8"
- 1 sm. red beet, sliced 1/8"

- 1 lrg. carrot, sliced 1/8"
- 2 tbsp. olive oil
- 1 tsp. fennel seeds, crushed
- ½ tsp. kosher salt
- 2 tbsp. fresh lemon juice
- 2 tsp. tarragon, fresh, chopped

Directions:

1.	Preheat oven to 450°F. Dry fish and place on a parchment-lined baking sheet. Arrange oranges and vegetables around it. Combine the oil, fennel seeds, salt, and pepper in a bowl. Drizzle oil over fish and vegetables.
2.	Bake for 10-12 minutes until the fish flakes. Sprinkle lemon juice and tarragon over top and serve.
3.	Place chicken back in skillet, put in the oven and bake until the chicken juices run clear. Remove from oven, sprinkle feta and dill over the top, then serve.

Breakfast - **Ricotta Spread w/ Fruit**

Servings: 4 -6

Nutritional Facts – Calories: 64 | Carbs: 3.5g | Fat: 8.3g | Protein: 7.1g

Ingredients:

- ♦ 1 cup ricotta, whole milk
- ♦ ½ cup almonds, sliced
- ♦ ¼ tsp. almond extract
- ♦ 1 tsp. honey
- ♦ Zest from orange

- ♦ For serving
- ♦ 2 pieces of bread
- ♦ Sliced peaches (or any fruit)
- ♦ almonds

Directions:

1.	Mix ricotta, almonds, and almond extract in a bowl until combined completely. Add extra almonds and drizzle honey over the top.
2.	Spread 1 spoon of mixture on each slice of bread and add peaches, almonds, and honey.

Lunch - **Chicken Kebabs pg.24**

Dinner - **Shrimp Piccata w/ Zucchini Noodles pg.34**

Breakfast - **Start Your Morning Right Grain Salad pg.10**

Lunch - **Hearts of Palm and Tomato Salad**

Servings: 4

Nutritional Facts – Calories: 133 | Carbs: 2.8g | Fat: 13.7g | Protein: .3g

Ingredients:

- 3 cups cherry tomatoes, halved
- 15 oz. can hearts of palm, drained, sliced
- ¼ cup red onion, sliced thin
- ¼ cup parsley, chopped
- ¼ cup olive oil
- 1 ½ tbsp. red wine vinegar
- 1 tsp. sugar
- 1 tsp. kosher salt
- ½ tsp. pepper

Directions:

1.	Combine all vegetables and fresh herbs together.
2.	In a separate bowl, combine the oil, vinegar, sugar, salt, and pepper and whisk until emulsified. Toss into vegetable mixture and serve.
3.	Serve sprinkled with chopped pistachios.

Dinner - **Roasted Stuffed Eggplant pg.48**

Breakfast - **Easy Muesli pg.12**

Lunch - **Garlic Steak w/ Warm Spinach pg.32**

Dinner - **Olive, Caper, and Lemon Chicken**

Servings: 6

Nutritional Facts – Calories: 147 | Carbs: 3.9g | Fat: 10.6g | Protein: 9.2g

Ingredients:

- 2 lemons, sliced ¼"
- ¼ cup olive oil, extra-virgin
- 6 chicken thighs, boneless
- 2 tbsp. flour, all-purpose
- 1 garlic clove, minced
- 1 cup chicken broth

- ¾ cup green olives
- ¼ cup capers
- 2 tbsp. butter
- 2 tbsp. parsley
- Kosher salt and pepper to taste

Directions:

1.	In a large skillet, heat 1 tbsp. of oil. Add in lemon slices and sear until browned. Remove and let sit. Season chicken and dredge in flour. Shake off excess. Add 1 ½ tbsp. of oil into the skillet and then place chicken thighs in skillet. Cook until golden brown on both sides. Remove from skillet and leave to rest with the lemon slices.
2.	Add in more olive oil and garlic. Cook until fragrant. Add in the broth capers and olives, as well as the chicken and lemons. Let simmer until broth reduces by half. Then, add butter and parsley. Cook for another minute and then season with salt and pepper. Remove from heat and serve.

Breakfast - **Baked Eggs w/ Avocado and Feta**

Servings: 2

Nutritional Facts – Calories: 282 | Carbs: 14.4g | Fat: 38.1g | Protein: 23.5g

Ingredients:

- ◆ 4 eggs
- ◆ 1 lrg. avocado
- ◆ Olive oil
- ◆ 3 tbsp. feta, crumbled
- ◆ Salt and pepper for taste

Directions:

1.	Break eggs into a ramekin and let come to room temperature.
2.	Preheat oven to 400°F and place gratin dishes on the baking sheet. Heat them in oven for 10 minutes.
3.	Cut avocado and slice. Remove dishes from oven and coat with olive oil. Place slices of avocado on the bottom of the dish and carefully pour two eggs in each.
4.	Sprinkle feta, salt and pepper over the top.
5.	Bake for 12-15 minutes and serve.

Lunch - **Slow Cooker Minestrone pg.50**

Dinner - **Pork Scaloppini w/ Lemon and Capers pg.16**

Breakfast - **Ricotta Spread w/ Fruit pg.84**

Lunch - **Lentil Patties w/ Mint Yogurt Sauce**

Servings: 4

Nutritional Facts – Calories: 413 | Carbs: 43g | Fat: 18g | Protein: 23g

Ingredients:

- 2 ½ tbsp. olive oil
- ½ cup onion, chopped
- 1 tbsp. garlic, minced
- ¾ cup rolled oats
- 2 tbsp. red wine vinegar
- 1 tsp. kosher salt
- ½ tsp pepper
- 2 lrg. eggs

- 1 pkg. brown lentils, steamed
- 2 cups arugula
- 2 cups baby spinach
- ¾ cup yogurt, Greek, plain
- 2 tbsp. fresh lemon juice
- 2 tbsp. mint, fresh, chopped
- 3 tbsp. pistachios, unsalted, chopped

Directions:

1.	Heat 1 ½ tsp. oil over medium heat in a large skillet. Add onion and garlic and cook until soft and fragrant. Combine this mixture with oats, 1 tbsp. vinegar, ¾ tsp. salt, pepper, eggs, and lentils into a food processor. Pulse until combined. Make into patties and let sit for a few minutes.
2.	Add 1 ½ tsp. of oil into skillet and cook patties in batches until both sides of each pattie are golden brown.
3.	Mix 1 tbsp. vinegar and 1 tbsp. oil and whisk together. Toss with spinach and arugula until coated.
4.	In a bowl, add together ½ tsp. salt, yogurt, juice, and mint.
5.	Lay a bed of greens and add the lentil cakes. Serve with chopped pistachios and yogurt sauce.

Dinner - **Bass w/ Tomatoes & Olives pg.37**

Breakfast - **Smoked Salmon & Poached Eggs on Toast pg.81**
Lunch - **Avocado Caprese Salad pg.54**
Dinner - **Pounded Chicken with Almond Paprika Vinaigrette**

Servings: 4

Nutritional Facts – Calories: 160 | Carbs: 4.4g | Fat: 15.8g | Protein: 2.1g

Ingredients:

- 4 chicken breasts, boneless, skinless
- ⅜ tsp. kosher salt
- ¼ tsp. pepper
- 3 tbsp. olive oil
- ¼ cup chicken stock, unsalted
- 1 garlic clove, minced
- 2 tbsp. water

- ¼ tsp. lemon zest
- 1 tbsp. lemon juice
- ¼ tsp. paprika, smoked
- ¼ tsp. Dijon mustard
- 2 tbsp. parsley, chopped
- 1 oz. green olives, chopped
- 2 tbsp. almonds, unsalted, roasted, chopped

Directions:

1.	Place chicken breast between a sheet of plastic wrap and pound until ¼ thick with meat mallet. Season both sides of the breast withsalt and pepper.
2.	Heat 1 ½ tsp. oil in a large skillet over medium-high heat. Add in chicken breasts and cook until brown on both sides. Remove when done and set aside.
3.	In the same skillet, add stock and reduce heat. Scrape up the browned bits and stir in 2 tbsp. of oil. Also, add in garlic and cook until fragrant. Then, add in ⅛ tsp. of salt, almonds, water, lemon juice, paprika, and mustard. Cook for a few minutes. Spoon the sauce over the chicken, sprinkle parsley and olives over the top, and serve.

Breakfast - **Pancakes w/ Greek Yogurt**

Servings: 6

Nutritional Facts – Calories: 258 | Carbs: 33g | Fat: 8g | Protein: 11g

Ingredients:

- 1 ¼ cup flour, all-purpose
- ¼ tsp. salt
- 2 tsp. baking powder
- 1 tsp. baking soda
- ¼ cup of sugar
- 3 tbsp. butter, unsalted, melted

- 3 eggs
- 1 ½ cups Greek yogurt, plain, non-fat
- ½ cup milk
- ½ cup blueberries (or other fruit)

Directions:

1.	Add flour, salt, baking powder, and baking soda to a large bowl and whisk until incorporated. In a separate bowl, add the sugar, melted butter, eggs, Greek yogurt, and milk. Whisk this mixture until combined fully. Slowly add the wet Ingredients to dry until fully combined. Let stand for 20 minutes.
2.	Heat the griddle and spray with no-stick spray. Use a ¼ cup measuring cup to pour batter onto the griddle. Cook until bubbles appear and then flip. Once fully browned on both sides, remove pancakes. Repeat the process until all the batter is gone.
3.	Top with more yogurt and fruit, then serve.

Lunch - **Grilled Eggplant Skillet pg.76**
Dinner - **Chicken Skillet w/ Bulgur pg.70**

Breakfast - **Frittata w/ Spinach and Artichoke pg.77**

Lunch - **Crock Pot Kale and Turkey Meatball Soup**

Servings: 10

Nutritional Facts – Calories: 446 | Carbs: 6.4g | Fat: 21.7g | Protein: 53.4g

Ingredients:

- ¼ cup milk
- 2 slices bread
- 1 lb. turkey, ground
- 1 med. shallot, chopped fine
- ½ tsp. nutmeg, fresh grated
- 1 tsp. oregano
- ¼ tsp. red pepper flakes
- Kosher salt and pepper to taste
- ½ cup parmesan, grated

- 2 tbsp. parsley, chopped
- 1 egg, beaten
- 1 tbsp. olive oil
- 8 cups chicken broth
- 15 oz. white beans, drained, rinsed
- 2 carrots, sliced
- ½ onion, chopped
- 4 cups kale

Directions:

1.	Add milk into the mixing bowl. Rip bread apart and soak in milk. Then add turkey, shallot, nutmeg, oregano, pepper flakes, salt, pepper, cheese, parsley, and egg. Mix well until combined. Use a scoop to form 1/2" meatballs.
2.	Heat the oil in a large skillet over medium-high heat. Then, sear meatballs in batches.
3.	Add broth, beans, and the vegetables into crockpot. Drop meatballs in and cook on low for 4 hours.
4.	Serve with red pepper flakes, parsley, and parmesan cheese sprinkled on top.

Dinner - **Greek Turkey Burgers pg.18**

Breakfast - **Baked Eggs w/ Avocado and Feta pg.87**
Lunch - **Hearts of Palm and Tomato Salad pg.85**
Dinner - **Pork and Orzo Mediterranean Style**

Servings: 6

Nutritional Facts – Calories: 372 | Carbs: 34g | Fat: 11g | Protein: 31g

Ingredients:

- 1 ½ lbs. pork tenderloin
- 1 tsp. pepper
- 2 tbsp. olive oil
- 3 qt. water
- 1 ¼ cup orzo
- ¼ tsp. salt
- 6 oz. baby spinach, fresh
- 1 cup grape tomatoes, halved
- ¾ cup feta, crumbled

Directions:

1.	Massage pepper into pork. Cut into 1" cubes. Heat oil over medium heat in a large skillet. Add pork and cook until done.
2.	In a Dutch oven, bring water to boil. Add in orzo and salt. Cook for 8 minutes, then add in spinach. Cook until orzo is al dente and spinach has wilted down. Drain.
3.	Add tomatoes to skillet with pork and heat all the way through. Mix with orzo and add cheese.

Breakfast - **Egg Muffins w/ Vegetable and Feta**

Servings: 6

Nutritional Facts – Calories: 114 | Carbs: 6g | Fat: 7g | Protein: 7g

Ingredients:

- 2 cups baby spinach, chopped
- ½ cup onion, chopped fine
- 1 cup tomatoes, chopped
- ½ cup kalamata olives, chopped
- 1 tbsp. oregano, fresh, chopped
- 2 tsp. sunflower oil
- 8 eggs
- 1 cup quinoa, cooked
- 1 cup feta, crumbled
- ¼ tsp. salt

Directions:

1.	Preheat oven to 350 ☐F. Oil the muffin tins.
2.	Heat skillet to medium heat and add in oil and onions. Cook until soft. Then, add in the tomatoes and cook for a minute. Now, add spinach and cook until wilted down. Remove from heat and add olives and oregano. Let sit.
3.	Add eggs into a bowl and whisk until well combined. Then, add in cooked quinoa, feta, and vegetables. Mix and add salt.
4.	Divide mixture evenly into muffin tin and bake for 30 minutes. Let cool and then serve.

Lunch - **Lentil Patties w/ Mint Yogurt Sauce pg.88**

Dinner - **Olive, Caper, and Lemon Chicken pg.86**

Breakfast – **Frittata w/ Asparagus, Mushroom, & Goat Cheese pg.6**

Lunch - **Turmeric Cauliflower Soup**

Servings: 6

Nutritional Facts – Calories: 149 | Carbs: 14g | Fat: 8g | Protein: 6g

Ingredients:

- ¼ cup pumpkin seeds, raw
- 1 tsp. cumin, ground
- 2 tbsp. thyme, fresh, chopped
- 6 garlic cloves, chopped
- 2 cups onion, sliced
- 2 tbsp. olive oil
- 1 tbsp. turmeric
- 1 tbsp. flour, all-purpose
- 2 ½ cups chicken stock, unsalted
- ½ tsp. kosher salt
- 1 sm. head cauliflower, cut into florets
- 2 tsp. rice vinegar
- 3 tsp. brown sugar, light
- ½ tsp. pepper
- ¼ cup sour cream, light
- 2 tbsp. chives, fresh, chopped

Directions:

1.	Mix pumpkin seeds, cumin, and 1 ½ tsp. of oil in a bowl. Then, heat a skillet over medium heat and add mixture. Toast the mixture until lightly browned. Remove the mixture and set it to the side.
2.	In a saucepan, heat 1½ tbsp. of oil over medium-high heat. Then, add onion, thyme, and garlic and cook until soft and fragrant. Then add turmeric and cook for another minute. Remove from heat.
3.	Whisk in a bowl ½ cup of stock and the flour until combined. Add salt, cauliflower, and rest of stock to the saucepan. Heat over high heat and bring to boil. Lower the heat and simmer for 15 minutes.
4.	Add this mixture into a food processor in batches and blend until smooth. Make sure to remove the center of the lid to release steam. When done, return to saucepan and stir in vinegar, sugar, and pepper. Cook for two minutes and then serve with pumpkin seeds, chives, and sour cream.

Dinner - **Parmesan Pesto Tilapia pg.39**

Breakfast - **Poached Eggs with Greens & White Beans pg.8**

Lunch - **Sun-Dried Tomato & Feta Couscous Salad pg.56**

Dinner - **Spicy Mussels**

Servings: 4

Nutritional Facts – Calories: 376 | Carbs: 26g | Fat: 10g | Protein: 38g

Ingredients:

- 1 tbsp. olive oil, extra-virgin
- 1 tbsp. butter, unsalted
- 2 tbsp. shallot, chopped fine
- 1 oz. prosciutto, diced
- 2 tsp. garlic, chopped
- ½ tsp. red pepper flakes
- 1 cup tomatoes, chopped
- ½ cup white wine, dry

- 1 tsp. sugar
- ⅜ tsp. kosher salt
- 2 lbs. mussels, scrubbed and debearded
- 2 tbsp. parsley, fresh, chopped
- 2 lemons, wedged
- Whole baguette, sliced and toasted

Directions:

1.	Heat olive oil and butter over medium-high heat in a Dutch oven. Then add shallot and prosciutto. Cook until shallots are soft and prosciutto is crisp. Add garlic and pepper flakes and cook until garlic is fragrant. Add tomatoes, wine, sugar, and salt and simmer
2.	Add mussels into the sauce. Cover and cook for appoximately 5 minutes until the mussels open. Serve in bowls with lemon wedges and crusty bread.

Breakfast - **Mediterranean Eggs**

Servings: 6

Nutritional Facts – Calories: 183 | Carbs: 11g | Fat: 11g | Protein: 9g

Ingredients:

- 1 ½ lrg. onions, sliced
- 1 tbsp. butter
- 1 tbsp. olive oil, extra-virgin
- 1 garlic clove, minced
- ⅓ cup sun-dried tomatoes, drained, sliced

- 6-8 lrg. eggs
- 3 oz. feta, crumbled
- Salt and pepper for taste
- ⅓ cup parsley, fresh, chopped fine

Directions:

1.	Heat butter and oil in a cast-iron skillet over medium heat. Add in onions and cook until soft. Reduce heat and let onions cook for another 5-10 minutes until a soft brown color. Then, add garlic and sun-dried tomatoes and let cook until fragrant.
2.	Spread the mix out until it is an even single layer on the bottom of the skillet. Crack eggs in skillet. Sprinkle the feta, salt, and pepper over the top. Cover skillet and cook for 10-15 minutes without removing the lid.
3.	Remove pan from heat and sprinkle parsley over top, then serve.

Lunch - **Tuna Melt w/ Olive Salsa pg.82**
Dinner - **Caprese Chicken pg.73**

Breakfast – **Avocado Toast Caprese Style pg.5**

Lunch - **Tomato Garlic Lentil Bowl**

Servings: 6

Nutritional Facts – Calories: 294 | Carbs: 49g | Fat: 3g | Protein: 21g

Ingredients:

- 1 tbsp olive oil
- 2 med. onions, chopped
- 4 garlic cloves, minced
- 2 cups dried lentils, brown, rinsed
- 1 tsp. salt
- ½ tsp. ginger, ground
- ½ tsp. paprika

- ¼ tsp. pepper
- 3 cups of water
- ¼ cup fresh lemon juice
- 3 tbsp. tomato paste
- ¾ cup Greek yogurt, fat-free, plain
- ⅓ cup cilantro, fresh, chopped

Directions:

1.	In a saucepan, heat oil over medium-high heat. Add onions and cook until soft. Then, add garlic and cook until it is fragrant. Stir in the lentils, seasoning, and water. Bring to a boil, then lower the heat and simmer covered for about 30 minutes.
2.	Mix in the lemon juice and tomato paste and heat through. Serve with yogurt and cilantro.

Dinner - **Honey Mustard Salmon pg.40**

Breakfast - **Start Your Morning Right Grain Salad pg.10**
Lunch - **Turmeric Cauliflower Soup pg.95**
Dinner - **Bruschetta Steak**

Servings: 4

Nutritional Facts – Calories: 280 | Carbs: 4g | Fat: 19g | Protein: 23g

Ingredients:

- 3 med. tomatoes, chopped
- 3 tbsp. basil, fresh, minced
- 3 tbsp. parsley, fresh, chopped
- 2 tbsp. olive oil
- 1 tsp. oregano, fresh, minced
- 1 garlic clove, minced
- ¾ tsp. salt
- 1 steak, flat-iron
- ¼ tsp. pepper
- ⅓ cup parmesan, grated

Directions:

1.	Combine tomatoes, basil, parsley, olive oil, oregano, and garlic. Add in ¼ tsp. salt and mix well. Then set to the side.
2.	Season beef with pepper and salt after cutting in four pieces. Heat a grill pan over medium heat. Then, grill the steak to preferred doneness. Let rest and then top with tomato mixture. Sprinkle parmesan over the top and serve.

The opinions and ideas of the author contained in this publication are designed to educate the reader in an informative and helpful manner. While we accept that the instructions will not suit every reader, it is only to be expected that the recipes might not gel with everyone. Use the book responsibly and at your own risk. This work with all its contents, does not guarantee correctness, completion, quality or correctness of the provided information. Always check with your medical practitioner should you be unsure whether to follow a low carb eating plan. Misinformation or misprints cannot be completely eliminated. Human error is real!

Picture: Blinovita Depositphotos // www.fieverr.com

Design: Oliviaprodesign

Printed in Poland
by Amazon Fulfillment
Poland Sp. z o.o., Wrocław